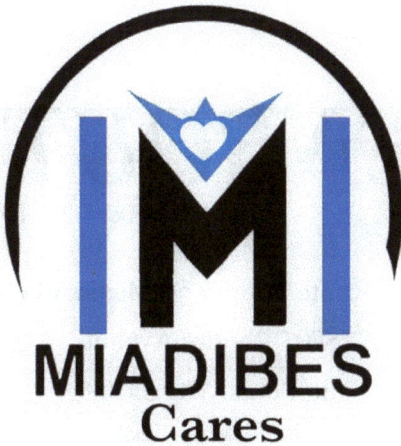

MIADIBES
Cares

Miadibes Cares

A Mission of Hope in the Blue Mountains

Kelly Mahfood

En Route Books and Media, LLC

Saint Louis, MO, USA

⊛*ENROUTE*
Make the time

Make the time

En Route Books and Media, LLC
5705 Rhodes Avenue
St. Louis, MO 63109

Cover credit: Kelly Mahfood
Copyright © 2025 Kelly Mahfood

ISBN-13: 979-8-88870-409-7
Library of Congress Control Number:
Available online at https://catalog.loc.gov

No part of this book may be reproduced, stored in a
retrieval system, or transmitted in any form, or by
any means, electronic, mechanical, photocopying,
or otherwise, without the prior written permission
of the author.

Acknowledgments

This book would not have been possible without the unwavering support, faith, and dedication of many incredible individuals and communities.

First and foremost, I want to thank God who is the fuel to this mission, the **Miadibes Cares team**—your passion, resilience, and commitment to service turned a vision into a movement. Each of you brought heart, skill, and spirit to every step of this mission, and I am deeply grateful for your partnership.

To our **generous donors**, thank you for believing in our cause and investing in the health and healing of communities beyond your own. Your contributions, both big and small, helped bring hope to Mount Prospect in ways words can never fully capture.

And to the **beautiful people of Mount Prospect**, thank you for welcoming us with open arms and open hearts. Your strength, hospitality, and grace reminded us why this work matters. You taught us just as much as we came to offer, and for that, we are forever humbled and inspired.

This journey has been one of purpose, growth, and deep connection. May the seeds we planted together continue to flourish.

With gratitude, **Kelly Mahfood**

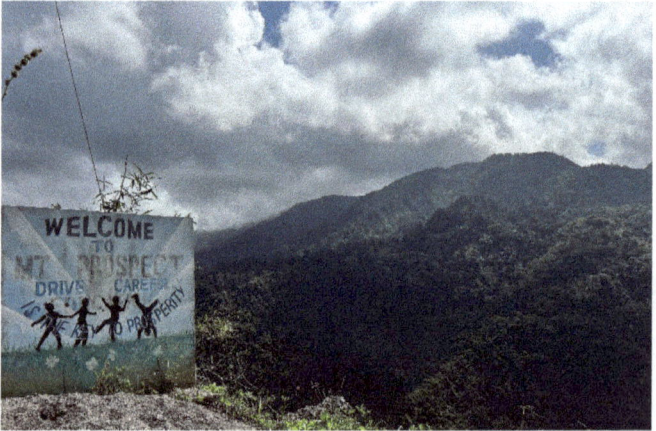

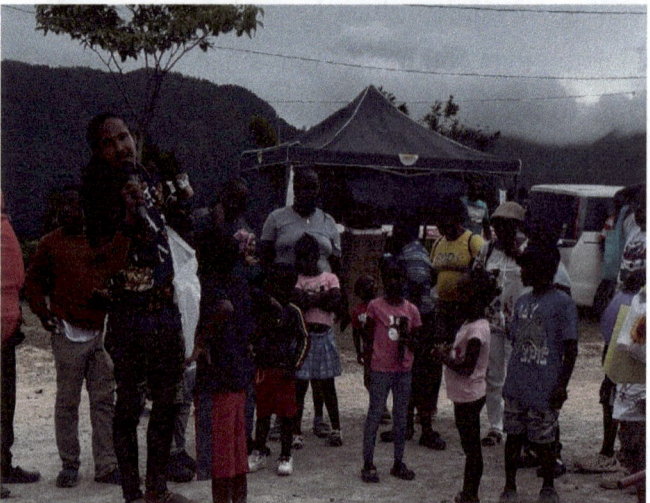

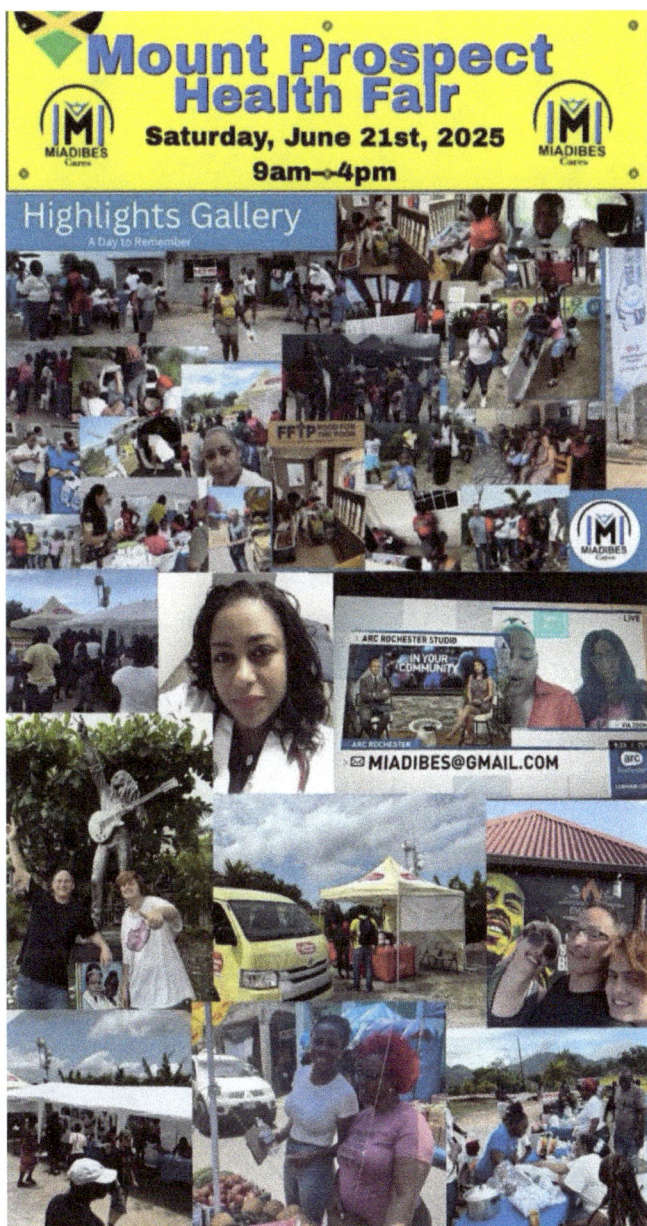

Mount Prospect Health Fair
Saturday, June 21st, 2025
9am-4pm

Highlights Gallery
A Day to Remember

Table of Contents

Foreword

"Let whoever is in charge keep this simple question in her head (not, 'how can I always do this right thing myself?), but 'how can I provide for this right thing to be always done?"

~Florence Nightingale~

Introduction

The Calling: How Miadibes Cares Was Born

Miadibes Cares was not born from a strategic plan or a polished pitch deck—it was born from a burden on my heart. As a nurse with over 25 years of experience, I've served countless patients in hospitals and clinics across the United States. But my mind and spirit have always remained tethered to Jamaica, the place of my roots, where so many families live without access to even the most basic healthcare services.

The seed was planted long before I ever realized I was being called to start a nonprofit. Each visit back home reminded me of the stark contrast between the healthcare systems I worked in, and the painful scarcity experienced in rural Jamaican communities like Mount Prospect. I'd see elders walking miles just to get their blood pressure checked, children going without dental care, and neighbors waiting months to address conditions that could be easily treated if only the resources were there.

In 2023, the vision began to crystalize. I had returned from a trip to St. Andrews with a heavy heart. That's when I began having real conversations—first with God, then with my family, and then with trusted colleagues and friends. The name "Miadibes Cares" came to me like a whisper, a blend of strength and compassion that echoed the mission I envisioned: to bring health, healing, and hope to Jamaica's most underserved populations.

With no budget, no sponsors, and no formal board, I began organizing. What started as a dream slowly turned into documents, meetings, and action plans. I leaned on my nursing background, my faith, and my community. I sent emails late at night, led Zoom meetings after work every Wednesday night, and packed barrels of medical supplies with my own hands.

The first major milestone was planning the Mount Prospect Health Fair for June 21, 2025. It was a bold goal—an entire health event in a remote mountain town, with screenings, medical consultations, education, and community celebration. And yet, through every setback, I felt confirmation that this was what I was meant to do.

Miadibes Cares isn't just an organization. It's a promise that no matter how remote or resource-limited a community may be, they are not forgotten. This is how our story began.

Why Mount Prospect? A Personal and Communal Connection

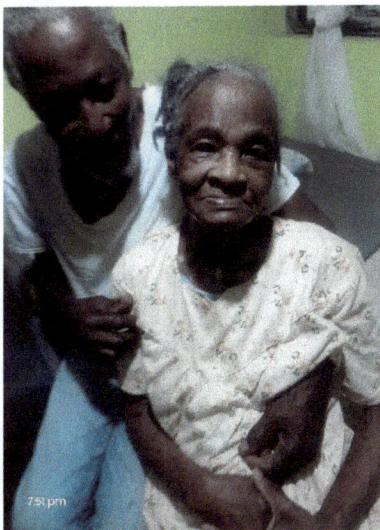

Mount Prospect is more than a pin on the map—it is the heartbeat of this mission. Nestled

Miadibes Cares –
Our First Mission

A New Beginning

Kelly Mahfood, Founder & CEO

This was the first mission of Miadibes Cares, a charity dedicated to health, healing, and hope in underserved rural communities in Jamaica. We are just getting started.

high in the Blue Mountains of St. Andrew, this rural community represents the soul of Jamaica: resilient, kind, and full of potential. But it also bears the burden of neglect, cut off from reliable healthcare due to limited infrastructure, sparse transportation, and economic hardship.

For me, Mount Prospect is deeply personal. It is where my family roots stretch back generations. I've walked its hilly roads, was taught in its school, and had conversations with elders who are disappointed that there are no clinic, no doctor, and no advocate. Every time I returned, I was reminded that while the landscape is lush, the resources are scarce.

Choosing Mount Prospect for the first health fair wasn't just about familiarity, it was about responsibility. I knew the people. I understood the needs. I felt the urgency. Mount Prospect stood as a symbol of countless other communities across Jamaica that had been left behind, and I wanted to shine a light here first.

Our mission in Mount Prospect has shown what's possible when compassion meets commitment. It proved that with enough heart, even the most remote communities can receive the dignity of care. And while Miadibes Cares is growing, our foundation will always be rooted in this village where it all began.

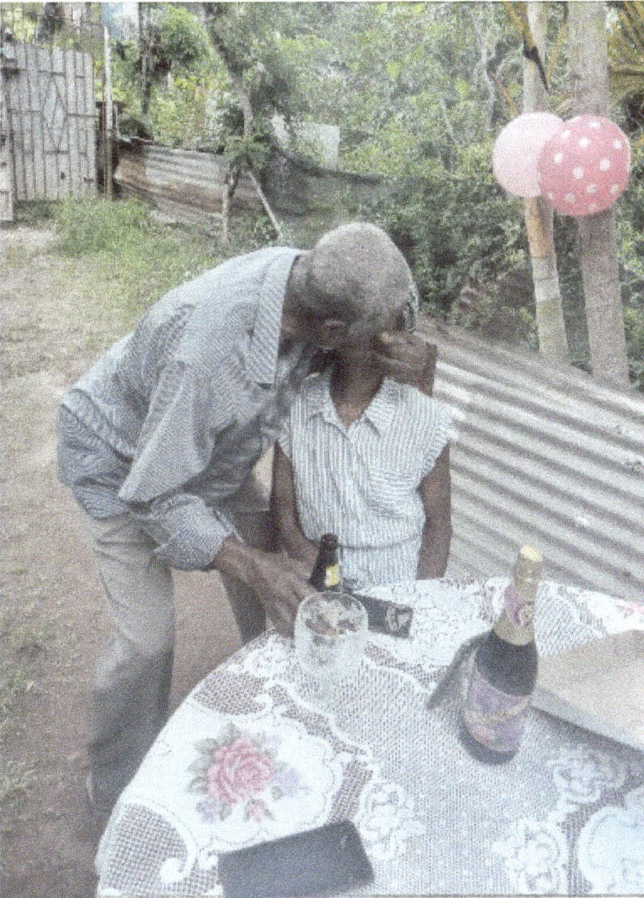

Part I

The Spark of Purpose

1

From Nurse to Founder

A Career of Service, A Heart for the Underserved

My nursing career has spanned over two decades, filled with long shifts, emotional triumphs, and countless lives touched. I've worked in trauma units, long-term care, skilled nursing, and clinical research. I've been a caregiver, an advocate, and a mentor. But through all the roles I've held, the most constant part of my identity has been service—serving people in their most vulnerable moments.

I've always been drawn to those who often go unseen—the elderly, the uninsured, the immigrants, the people living paycheck to paycheck. I found fulfillment not just in procedures and protocols, but in listening, holding a hand, and reminding someone they mattered. My heart has always beat strongest for the underserved.

Recognizing the Healthcare Crisis in Rural Jamaica

It was during my visits to Jamaica that I began to fully grasp the depth of the healthcare crisis facing rural communities. What I saw wasn't just inconvenient, it was heartbreaking. Entire communities without access to a nearby clinic. Children with untreated skin infections. Adults unaware of their blood pressure or blood sugar levels. Pregnant women with no access to prenatal care, young people dying from upper respiratory infections due to lack of knowledge and treatment. My very own uncle "Culture Rat" died in 2023 of pneumonia that was not treated in time. He became short of breath and while his body lost oxygen, he became delirious and combative. He did not know nor understood what was happening to him. By the time someone noticed how ill he was, it was too late. Not long after getting to the hospital in Kingston, he passed away from respiratory distress. I can share my comments on the hospital's role in this mishap, but I'll save that for later. He was being combative and kept removing his oxygen mask, that shows he did not understand what was going on. I hope and pray the hospital system will become a safer and better place for the sick and underprivileged people of Jamaica.

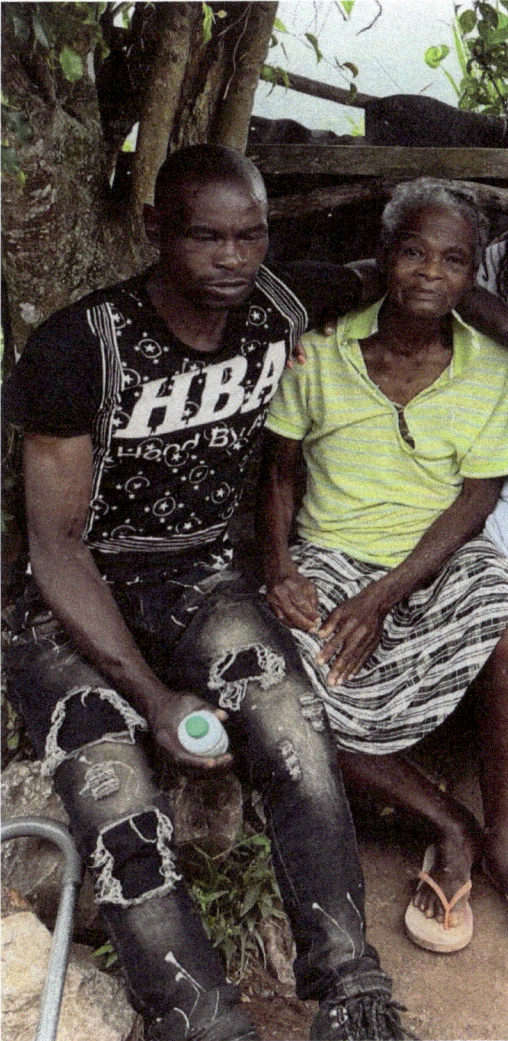

R.I.P. Donavan Edwards AKA "Culture Rat"
June 11th, 1970, ~ May 2023

The more I visited, the more I couldn't unsee it. While Jamaica has talented doctors and nurses, the resources are too often concentrated in urban centers, leaving remote villages behind. Public transportation is limited. Pharmacies are far away. Health education is lacking. And systemic neglect has made the situation feel normal to those living in it.

I knew I couldn't fix everything—but I also knew I couldn't walk away. This awareness became the foundation of Miadibes Cares. I wanted to create a bridge—between healthcare providers and the people who needed them most. Between my nursing experience and the villages of my childhood. Between compassion and action.

This chapter, like the beginning of Miadibes Cares itself, marks a shift—from a nurse serving one patient at a time to a founder advocating for an entire community.

2

Building the Vision

Naming the Mission: "Miadibes Cares"

The name "Miadibes Cares" came to me not from a brainstorming session, but from a spiritual nudge—one of those moments when inspiration feels divine. The name holds meaning: "Miadibes" is a powerful word drawn from personal significance and strength. Striving, to be the best, Being Jamaican and standing on pride and strength, while "Cares" captures the spirit of compassion and action that drives everything we do. Using Miadibes with other life interests for a long time now like my pepper sauce; Miadibes Peppa Sauce and my Miadibes Black cakes, continuing the name with a caring spin on it just made sense. It wasn't just about naming a nonprofit—it was about declaring our purpose to the world.

In that name, I saw our entire mission: to care for those who feel forgotten. To show up in places that others overlook. To remind people that their lives matter, and they deserve access to health, healing, and hope.

Conversations That Planted the Seeds

Before Miadibes Cares ever launched, there were conversations—many quiet, honest talks with my family, my faith circle, my friends, and my colleagues. Some were filled with excitement, others with concern. "That's a lot to do," they'd say. Or "How will you pay for it?", or "Maybe you should wait until your finances are better." I didn't always have answers, but I had conviction.

I remember long phone calls, Zoom Meetings, and Whatsapp video calls. I asked questions, listened deeply, and started shaping the idea in a way that others could grasp. Those early conversations helped me realize that I wasn't alone. I was surrounded by people who believed in the mission—even when they didn't fully understand it.

In those moments Miadibes Cares began to take form—not just in my mind, but in the hearts of others.

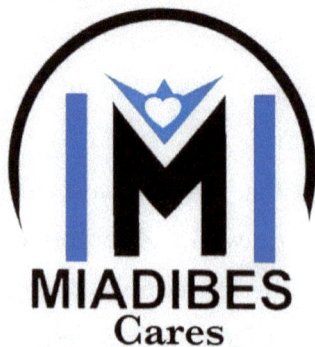

MIADIBES
Cares

Early Fears and Faith

Launching a nonprofit from the ground up is no small task. I had fears: fear of failure, fear of not being taken seriously, fear of letting people down. I wondered if I was too late, too underfunded, too ambitious. But faith overruled fear, every time.

My faith reminded me that purpose doesn't require perfection, it requires obedience. So, I kept moving. I leaned into prayer, leaned on my support system, and reminded myself of the people in Mount Prospect who were still waiting for care.

That faith became my fuel. It gave me the strength to push through doubt and keep building the vision, one step at a time.

3

Registering a Dream

Nonprofit Formation: Navigating the U.S. and Jamaican Systems

Turning Miadibes Cares into an official non-profit organization was one of the most complex chapters of the journey. In the United States, it meant researching 501(c)(3) requirements, drafting bylaws, filing articles of incorporation, and ensuring tax compliance. It also meant opening a business account, creating a board, and laying the groundwork for ethical stewardship. While working on legitimizing this organization, I was blessed enough to have mentorship from my cousin Dr. Sebastian Mahfood of WCAT Radio where Miadibes Cares is able to operate under their umbrella in the mean time until we get our own 501(c)(3) and Cornell Bunting of EHAS (Everyone Has A Story) who share knowledge and support.

In Jamaica, the process is even more nuanced. I must navigate different legal structures, connect with local attorneys, and begin the early steps of establishing charitable registration. Every document requires careful translation between countries, systems, and expectations. It feels like starting a business and building a ministry—at the same time, on two different islands.

Legal, Financial, and Logistical Hurdles

The paperwork alone was overwhelming. I spent nights reading IRS manuals and days emailing government offices. I learned how to draft resolutions, submit compliance forms, and respond to requests for clarification. There were delays, missed emails, and frustrating red tape.

Financially, I had to front many of the early expenses myself—paying for incorporation fees, purchasing supplies, and covering travel. Fundraising didn't come overnight. I had to learn how to write proposals, approach donors, and explain the vision in ways that moved hearts and opened wallets.

Then there were the logistics: setting up secure storage for medical supplies, navigating customs regulations, and building communication systems for a growing team of volunteers. Every small success felt like a miracle—and every obstacle was a chance to grow stronger.

Learning While Doing

There was no manual for this. I had never started a nonprofit before. But I believed in the mission so deeply that I was willing to learn everything I didn't know.

I enrolled in webinars, joined nonprofit forums, asked questions, and listened closely to mentors. Each mistake taught me something important. Each success gave me the courage to keep going.

In the end, Miadibes Cares was not built by perfect planning it was built by perseverance. We were learning while doing, fueled by a vision that was too important to delay. And every step we took brought us closer to serving the people who needed us most.

Part II

Planning the Impossible

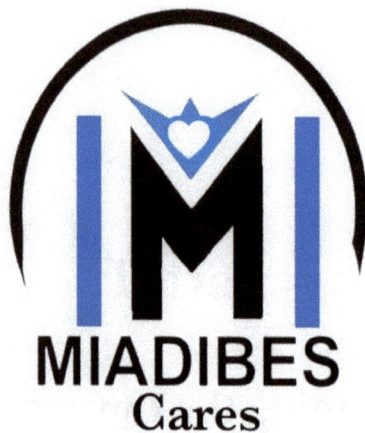

MIADIBES
Cares

SATURDAY, JUNE 21, 2025
9AM TO 4PM

Mount Prospect Health Fair

A proposal to for organizing a Health Fair
for *the rural area of Mount Prospect, St. Andrews, Jamaica*

PRESENTED BY

Kelly Mahfood

4

Mount Prospect:
A Community in Need

Health Disparities in Rural Jamaica

Rural Jamaica is rich in culture, community, and resilience—but when it comes to healthcare, the disparities are undeniable. For decades, systemic issues have created a gaping divide between urban centers and remote mountain villages like Mount Prospect. In Kingston, hospitals are buzzed with activity, and medical specialists are accessible. But just an hour away (Depending on traffic and considering the road conditions), residents of places like Mount Prospect, Mount Airy, and Mount Pleasant often go years without seeing a physician.

High blood pressure, diabetes, and untreated injuries are common. Many people rely on home remedies or simply go without care altogether, and some even die. The absence of transportation infrastructure, limited access to pharmacies, and a lack of continuous health education all compound the problem. For expectant mothers, aging adults, and those with chronic illnesses, the cost of isolation can be fatal. Many people are left alone while their children and relatives are living abroad, some who have turned their backs on their families and country. While the elderly become older and alone with progressive illnesses that cripples them on their properties due to bad roads and lack of transportation.

This is the silent crisis Miadibes Cares set out to confront. Our mission is about more than hosting events—it's about disrupting generational neglect with sustainable, community-based solutions.

Meeting the People, Hearing Their Stories

The planning began with listening.

Before we selected a location or ordered a single blood pressure cuff, we walked through Mount Prospect, met with families, and sat with elders under mango trees. We heard about missed diagnoses, long walks to Golden Springs or Stony Hill just to get to a clinic, and prayers whispered for loved ones who never received the care they needed. These stories weren't just emotional, they were clarifying.

One woman shared how she waited over a year for a follow-up on a CT scan. A man showed us his prescription papers for x-rays and bloodwork he could not afford to get done. A neighbor spoke of how kids miss school because of preventable illnesses that were going untreated. My very own grandfather (Oneson is his name) who cut his foot on my grandmother's wheelchair and told no one until it was severely infected that he couldn't walk, Experiencing a medical emergency on a video call to my grandparents, watching my grandmother passing out in the bathroom and knowing we don't have the option to call 911 (119 in Jamaica), there are no services of that sorts in their area. I had to call someone I know who drove them to Stony Hill Doctor's office where she was treated for elevated blood Pressure and given new prescriptions, A relative who's child is blinking uncontrollably for months and unable to afford to get an eye exam done. Their words and situations weren't complaints—they were calls for help wrapped in resilience.

Those situations became the foundation of our planning. Every smile, every tear, and every handshake reminded us that this mission wasn't about charity, it was about justice. I was ready to grab my stethoscope and blood pressure cuff and sit right there in the town square and check everyone's blood pressure.

Site Selection: UB Church & Basic School

Finding the right location to host our first health fair was both a logistical and spiritual decision. We needed somewhere accessible, familiar, and trusted by the community. The Mount Prospect United Brethren (UB) Church and the nearby Basic School stood out immediately.

These two institutions have long been pillars of the community—places where my own relatives gather not just for worship or learning, but for support. They're centrally located, with open grounds and modest facilities that could be transformed into makeshift clinics, Vision Screening areas, triage stations, and even Registration and survey waiting space.

With the church's blessing and the school's co-operation, we secured the grounds. Volunteers helped measure space and envision how we could bring modern healthcare screening to these historic grounds—if only for a day.

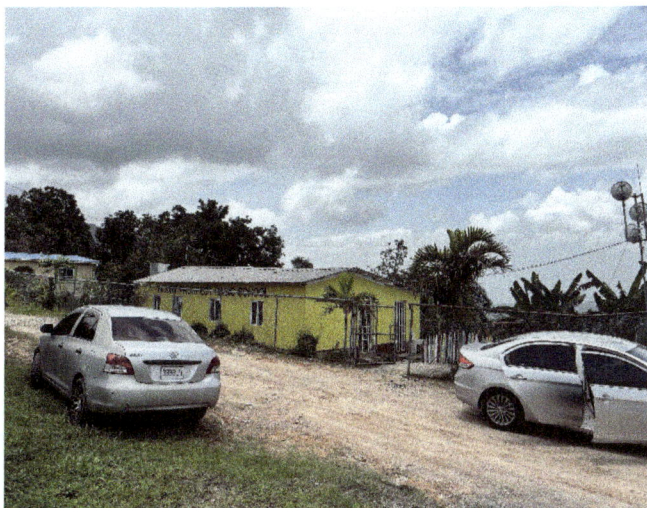

The moment we confirmed the location, the impossible began to feel tangible. We weren't just planning an event—we were preparing to transform lives in the very heart of the community.

5

The Proposal That Made It Real

Crafting the Official Plan

After securing the location, it was time to formalize our dream. We needed more than good intentions—we needed a clear and compelling proposal to guide our next steps and engage partners. I sat down at my laptop, opened a blank document, and typed the words: *"Proposal for Sponsorship & Support: Mount Prospect Health Fair."* It wasn't just a title. It was a statement of belief in what we were about to do.

The document outlined every detail of our vision: what we hoped to provide, who we aimed to serve, and how we would execute it. We laid out sections on logistics, staffing, supplies, volunteer coordination, and community involvement. We included stories and context of why Mount Prospect was chosen. The proposal wasn't just paperwork—it was our blueprint of purpose.

Objectives, Budget, and What We Hoped to Achieve

We dreamed big but planned smart. Our objectives were threefold: (1) provide free health screenings and wellness education to at least 200 community members, (2) build partnerships with healthcare professionals and local organizations, and (3) create a replicable model that could be used in other underserved communities.

Our budget included everything from tents and medical equipment to meals for the local residents, volunteers and transportation stipends. We knew the road wouldn't be easy, but we believed that transparency, organization, and prayer would open the doors we needed. Every dollar mattered. Every line item reflected a commitment to impact.

Sending the First Sponsorship Letters

The day we sent our first sponsorship letters was terrifying and exhilarating. I reached out to friends, family, businesses, churches, and medical professionals with a message that was part invitation, part plea: *"Join us in bringing healing to Mount Prospect."*

A lot didn't respond. Some said they'd think about it. But others—oh, the others! They said yes. They donated money, supplies, time, and trust. With each new supporter, our confidence grew. We weren't in this alone. This wasn't just my calling anymore. It was becoming a shared mission.

And with every signature, every donation, and every encouraging message, the impossible came closer to reality.

6. Fundraising, Faith, and a Few Barrels

$900 and a Mountain to Climb

Our first real budget total was sobering: $900 in the bank and a full-scale health fair to pull off in a remote village on a mountainside. We didn't have sponsors lined up. We didn't have corporate backers or grants. All we had was belief that if we moved forward in faith, the rest would follow.

But faith, as we quickly learned, requires action.

Every cost added up: shipping, medical supplies, tents, food, transport, printing, and lodging. Just getting things from Atlanta to Kingston, and then up the mountain to Mount Prospect, was a challenge. I was happy to find out that the 77-gallon barrel can fit into my back seat so going to purchase them one at a time was tedious but not as stressful as what I had to go through before knowing this. I had to rent a pick-up truck and drive it all the way to the warehouse which is one hour away from me. The drive was treacherous and shaky. Not being skilled at driving large vehicles stressed me out. When we ran the numbers, the mountain felt even steeper. But we didn't back down. We rolled up our sleeves and got creative.

Packing Barrels, Shipping Woes, and Customs Costs

Packing the barrels became its own adventure. I requested assistance from family members and friends, but everyone lived so far apart that it became difficult for others to come by to help to sort out the donations. I had to start even if I had to pack it by myself—blood pressure cuffs, glucometers, hygiene kits, coloring books, crayons, personal care items, even feminine products. I packed with care and prayed over each barrel, knowing the items would touch hands and hearts that truly needed them.

Then came the shipping drama. Delays. Miscommunications. Unexpected fees. Customs clearance was another beast entirely. We paid duties on items that had been donated out of love. We navigated paperwork, receipts, and endless phone calls to make sure the barrels didn't just arrive—but got released on time. Which didn't happen. Issues with investigations at the Jamaican Wharf delayed my shipment from being unloaded off the ship for two weeks. I had never known stress like waiting for your health fair supplies to be "cleared" from a warehouse in Kingston days before your event. Spending seven hours at the wharf was an experience. I had to pay extra fees to the shipping company just because I didn't use my entire first name. They called it a name change fee. Then I had to pay the same fee to the customs department for the same issue. Redundant fees got me feeling like I was being scammed.

Still, with God and persistence, the barrels made it to Mount Prospect.

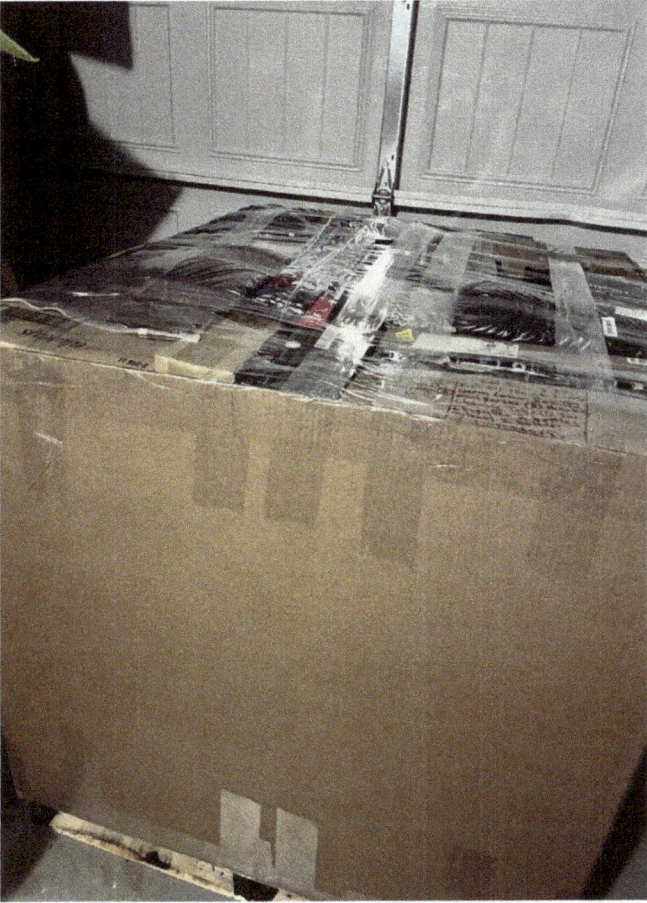

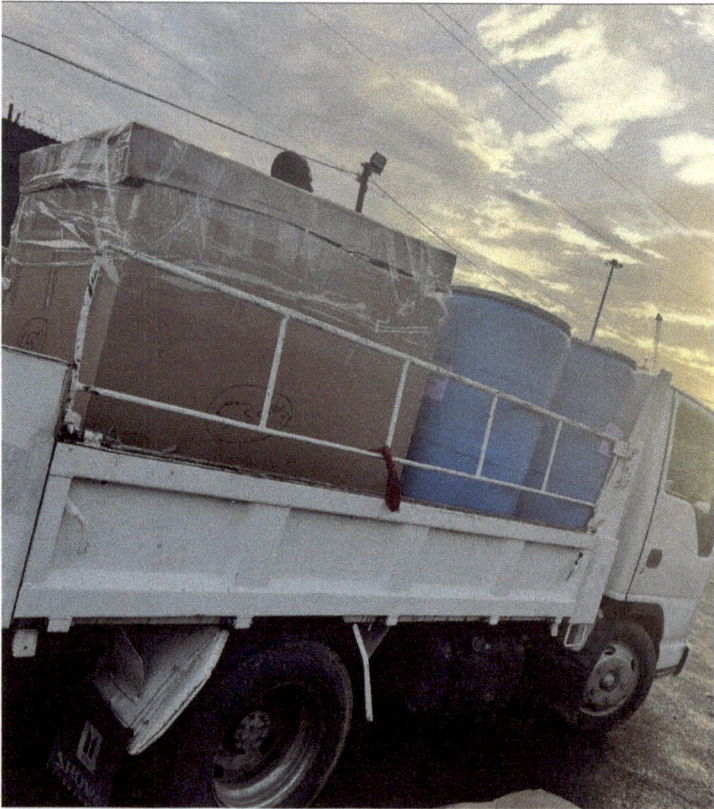

**Picking up the shipment from the wharf just days
before the health fair**

Creative Fundraising: GoFundMe, Gala, Raffle, Ice Cream Truck

With limited funds and mounting expenses, we turned to the community. We launched a Go-FundMe and began telling our story publicly sharing the vision, the stakes, and the people we hoped to serve. Donations trickled in. Then poured in. Some gave $10. Others gave hundreds. Every gift was fuel for our fire. But we didn't stop there. Every idea was on the table. Every dollar raised felt like one more step closer to Mount Prospect. Thanks to WCAT Radio for being our umbrella and allowing us to have those who donated to have that money be tax deductible through their organization using their 501(c)(3) number.

People bought in—not just financially, but emotionally. They believed in what we were building. They saw the photos, read the testimonies, and understood this was more than a health fair. It was a mission.

And with each barrel, and blessing, Miadibes Cares took one more step toward becoming real.

Part III

Building a Movement

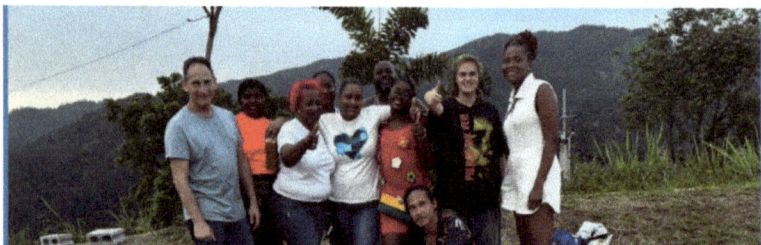

Our Amazing Volunteers

Special thanks to:
- Javina Francis (Registration Lead) – flawless coordination!
- Dr. Sebastian Mahfood, Dr. Stephanie Mahfood, & Eva for being such a blessing to this mission.
- Shannon, Bruce, Annette, Joy, Mervin, Debbie, Mrs. Wallace, Ms. Collie, Ms. Hall, Chef O'Niel, Mr. Pampaz, Stephanie Marley of Wake Up Jamaica
- Pastor Jermaine Campbell of CUBIC, Mount Prospect
- Patrick, The Sound System folks, Cory, D from Trelawny
- Javar AKA Chin the Man (Driver, Spiderman and all around our go to guy)
- Gadafy aka "Daddy" – MVP clean-up and fun loving attitude!

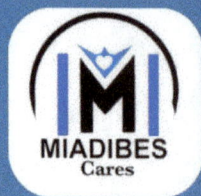

7

Volunteers & Visionaries

Creating the Core Team

The dream of Miadibes Cares could not have been realized without the people who stood behind it. Our core team came together not through job postings or formal interviews but through heartfelt conversations, shared passion, and a mutual sense of calling. Friends became team leaders, family members became logistics managers, and strangers turned into mission partners. What united us was the belief that something beautiful could happen in Mount Prospect.

Weekly Zoom Meetings, WhatsApp Updates, and Rallying the Diaspora

Our operations hub was virtual—but full of heart. Weekly Zoom calls became a rhythm, where ideas sparked, tasks were assigned, and milestones were celebrated. WhatsApp chats ran day and night, filled with images of donated supplies, spreadsheet updates, and prayers for customs clearance.

We reached out to the Jamaican diaspora—nurses, doctors, artists, and business professionals who had roots in Jamaica and a willingness to give back. Slowly, momentum built. It wasn't just a mission anymore—it was a movement.

Recognizing Fatigue, Reigniting Commitment

But building a mission from scratch is no small feat. As the weeks rolled on, fatigue set in. Some team members were balancing full-time jobs, family responsibilities, and health challenges. We saw signs of burnout—and we named it. We paused to breathe, to pray, to check in. And when we needed to, we reignited the fire with stories of why we started, pictures of the people we'd serve, and reflections of the difference we knew we could make.

8

Partnerships, Sponsors & Surprises

Scotiabank, Grace Kennedy, WCAT, and Others

The road to sponsorships was humbling. We reached out to large corporations— Jamaican Teas (Caribbean Dreams), CB Chicken, Comprehensive Eyecare, Wake Up Jamaica, UWI Nursing Program, Food For The Poor, Scotiabank, Grace Kennedy, WCAT Radio, and others. A few responded generously. Others didn't respond at all. But every "yes" we received reminded us that people and companies saw the value in what we were doing.

These partners contributed in various ways— financial gifts, bottled water, tents, snacks, printing services, Over the Counter Medications, and even staffing support. We were grateful for every ounce of help.

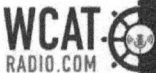

WCAT RADIO.COM LOVE LIFTS UP WHERE KNOWLEDGE TAKES FLIGHT

Corporate Giving vs. Community Goodwill

Some of the most profound support came not from big brands but from everyday people—social media friends purchased items from our Amazon Registry, Mount Prospect CUBIC Pastor assisted with getting paperwork officially notarized for requesting services from companies, and loved ones and strangers donated whatever they could. There was something incredibly pure about community-driven goodwill. It was personal. It was passionate. It was powerful.

We learned that impact isn't just about corporate backing. Sometimes the most transformational support comes from the people with the least to give—but the biggest hearts.

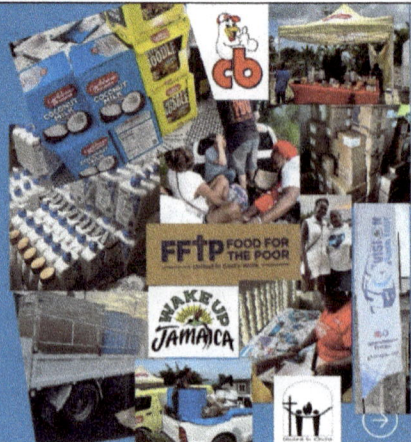

With Heartfelt Gratitude

Together we were a success

We extend our deepest thanks to every volunteer, donor, sponsor, and attendee who made our very first Miadibes Cares Health Fair a tremendous success.

Lessons Learned from Chasing Sponsorships

We also learned to manage expectations. Not every promising lead turn into a sponsor. Not every big name will see your vision. And that's okay. We learned to pivot, stay faithful to the mission, and keep building, one relationship at a time.

9

Event Week: Chaos and Calling

Traveling to Jamaica, Final Logistics

By the time our team boarded planes for Jamaica, the months of planning felt like a blur. There were still last-minute forms to print (Which was an exhausting chore), supplies to pack, and emails to send. Coordinating transport from Kingston to the Blue Mountains required patience, flexibility, and a little divine intervention from our faithful and reliable driver Javar. He is such a blessing to have on the team.

I stayed in the guest bedroom of my grandparents' house. Signals were difficult in that area, and I had to travel to Kingston daily to hotels just to use their Wi-Fi. I set myself up in a comfortable area and ordered food and drinks from the bar. Shirley Temples was my drink of choice during this venture. Sometimes I recruited a family member to come with me. We would work hard to reach possible sponsors and donors for hours while enjoying a beautiful and cool atmosphere. When we were ready to go, I would call our driver and head on to the next activity.

Volunteers trickled in—some from the U.S., others from different parts of Jamaica in the Kingston and St. Andrews areas. Accommodations were secured, meals planned, and a final sweep of the Mount Prospect site was done. Time was extremely valuable, and I was able to record a short video at the site to share with the team and with our social media.

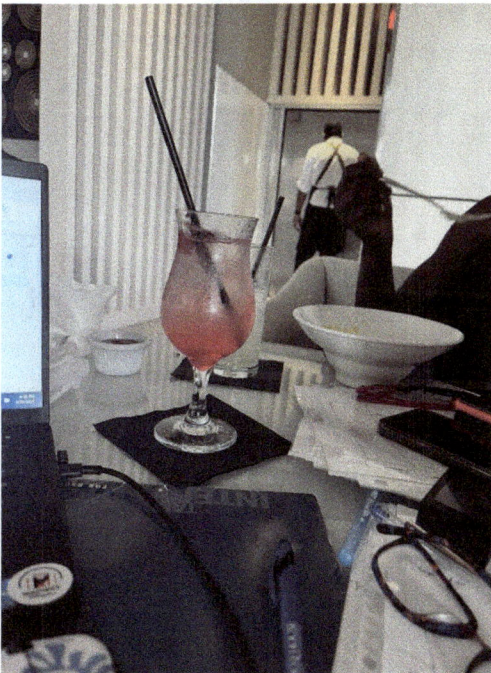

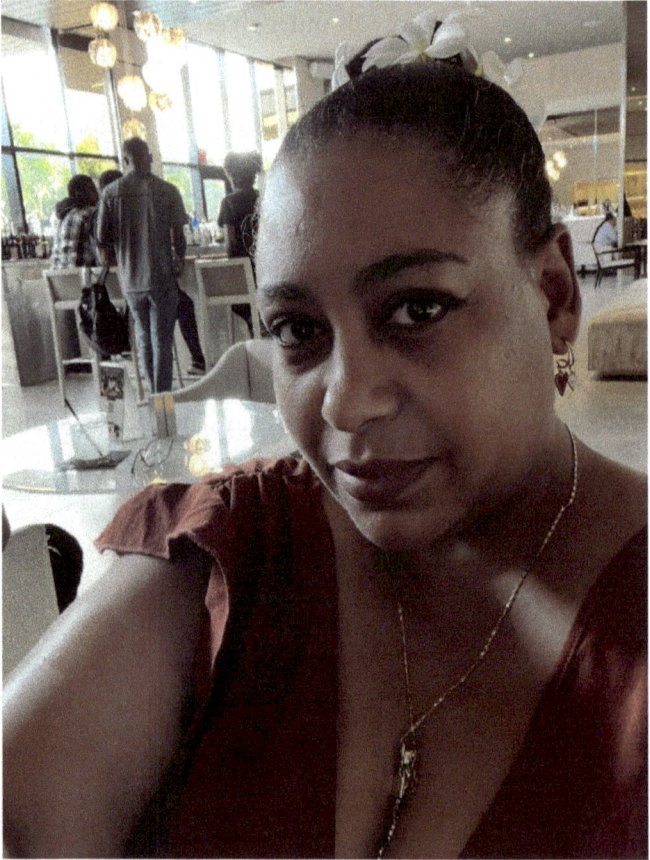

Vision Screening, Nursing Volunteers, Medical Tents

Event day came like a sunrise—sudden and full of beauty. The sun came out early and the skies were clear. The beautiful Blue Mountain tops were touched with small patches of cloudy mists, setting up the medical tent was its own monster, we welcomed the local residents with smiles, music, and hope. Our nursing volunteers from UWI, Mona wore custom shirts from their school, and each person knew their role—from registration to screening, consultation to kids' activities.

It was a symphony of service.

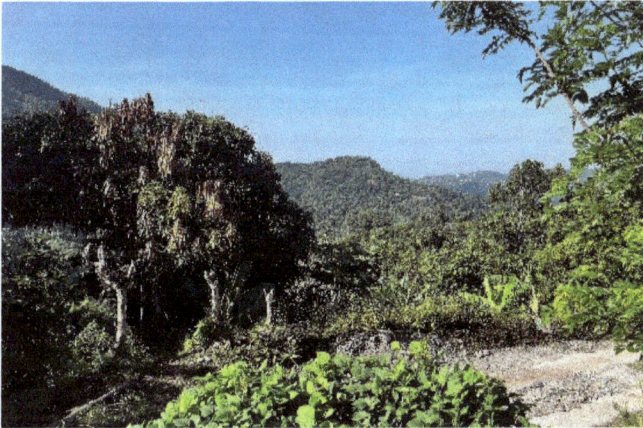

Behind the Scenes Heroes
Silent Stars Who Made It Happen

- Mr. Pampaz – transport support
- Gadafy & the clean-up crew
- Pastor Jermaine Campbell & the CUBIC, Mount Prospect Church
- Principal Mrs. Wallace & the Basic School
- Dr. Sebastian and Stephanie Mahfood - All around support
- Maxine Hamilton AKA Rudie - Donor outreach MVP
- Donors

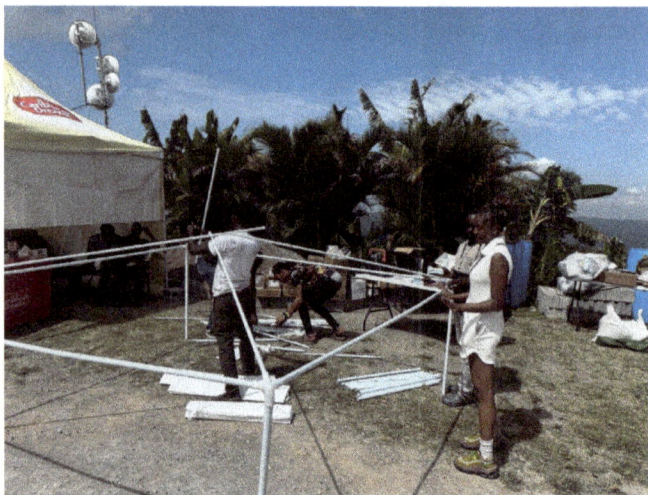

Overcoming Last-Minute Crises

Of course, it wasn't without chaos. We faced misplaced items, the tent was difficult to assemble, a sudden rain shower with heavy winds almost blew away the tent, and a minor rift between some kids. But nothing could stop us. We pivoted and waited out the rain inside the church and tents, counseled the kids with their parents and pressed on.

What we saw that day was the culmination of every vision board, every late-night meeting, every dollar raised, and every faith-filled step. The chaos became sacred. The calling came alive.

Part IV

The Mountaintop Moment

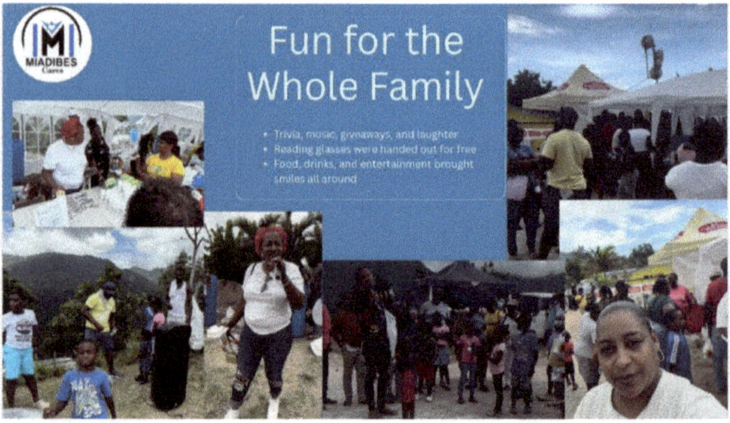

Community came together for a good cause

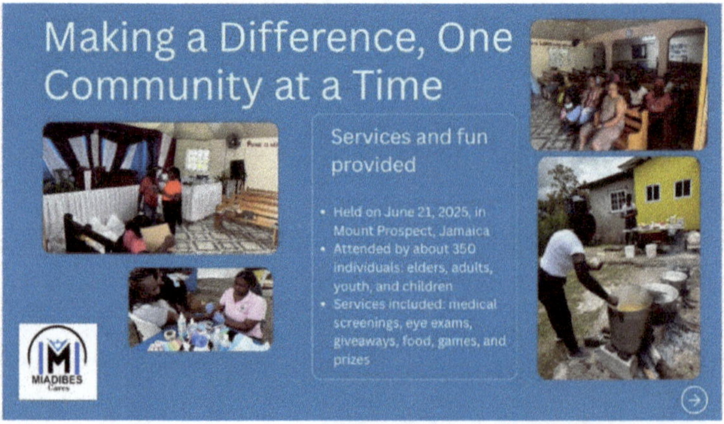

10

June 21, 2025 – The Health Fair

The morning of June 21, 2025, began with bird-song and nervous excitement. From sunrise, the team was on-site setting up tents, arranging tables, unloading supplies, and coordinating traffic flow. The music started, the community began arriving, and the atmosphere felt electric with purpose.

Screening stations were humming with activity—blood pressure checks, diabetes testing, eye exams were being done on the veranda of the church, and health consultations. Volunteers moved swiftly and kindly, creating a welcoming environment. Children were given refreshment, tote bags with supplies, coloring books, and bubbles to keep them engaged while their parents were seen.

People shared their stories—some had walked miles to get there from their farms, others had never had their blood pressure checked before. There was a man who learned he had high blood pressure and was educated in our consultation area on what to do next. Free reading glasses were given out to anyone who needed them. Some came late but we were prepared and had supplies to give out to the late comers.

We collected data—over 300 attendees, hundreds of screenings completed, and every family walked away with something in their gift bags: medication, toys, personal supplies, a resource, and simply the feeling that they mattered.

The energy was contagious—joy, health, and healing flowed freely under the Jamaican sun on top of the Blue Mountains.

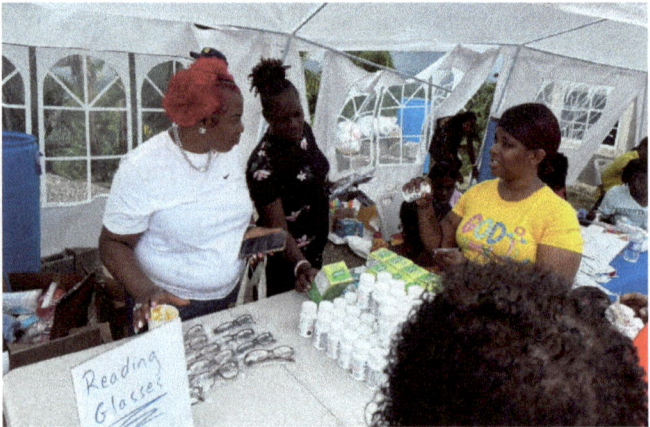

11

Looking Ahead:
The Vision Continues

The work of Miadibes Cares did not end with the health fair—it only deepened. As we returned to our homes across Jamaica and the United States, our minds were already spinning with ideas for the future.

One of the most anticipated milestones ahead is the **Miadibes Cares Awards Gala**, scheduled for June 12th, 2026. This black and white attire formal gathering will honor the volunteers, donors, and community partners who made this mission possible as well as honoring all works of charity throughout the diaspora. It will be a time of reflection and recognition, celebrating not only what was accomplished but what is still to come.

Planning is underway for the **Second Annual Mount Prospect Health Fair**, with lessons learned guiding our way. We are expanding our partnerships, refining logistics, and increasing outreach so we can serve even more families in 2026.

Most importantly, our team is growing stronger. New volunteers have expressed interest, more sponsors are joining the mission, and our faith remains unwavering. We move forward with gratitude in our hearts and the mountain still in our vision.

Mount Prospect was just the beginning.

Part V

Beyond the Fair

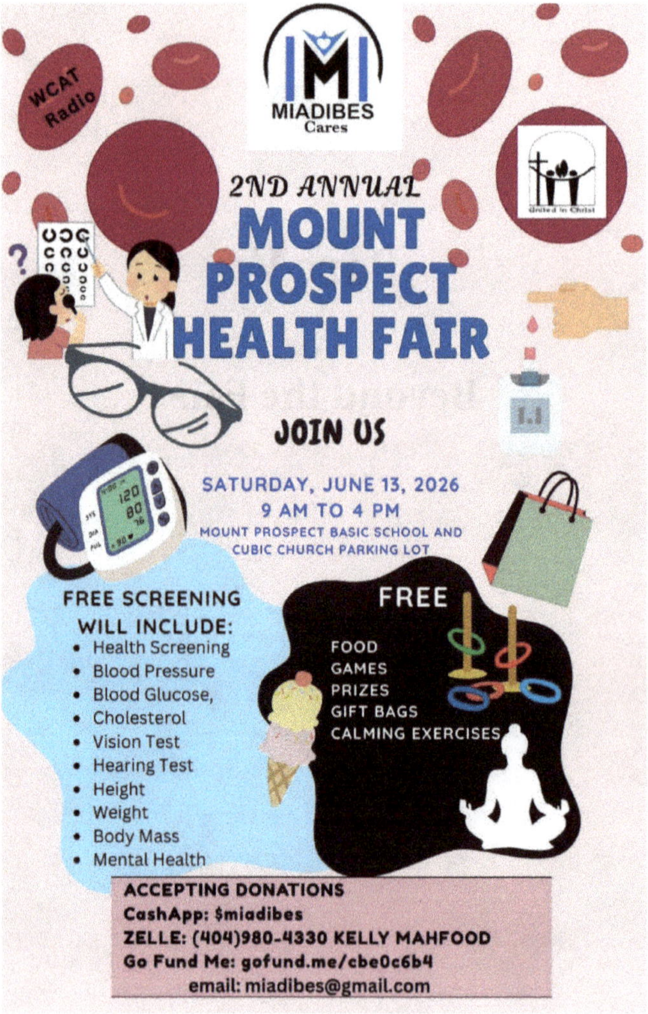
WCAT Radio
MIADIBES Cares
United in Christ
2ND ANNUAL
MOUNT PROSPECT HEALTH FAIR
JOIN US
SATURDAY, JUNE 13, 2026
9 AM TO 4 PM
MOUNT PROSPECT BASIC SCHOOL AND CUBIC CHURCH PARKING LOT
FREE SCREENING WILL INCLUDE:
• Health Screening
• Blood Pressure
• Blood Glucose,
• Cholesterol
• Vision Test
• Hearing Test
• Height
• Weight
• Body Mass
• Mental Health
FREE
FOOD
GAMES
PRIZES
GIFT BAGS
CALMING EXERCISES
ACCEPTING DONATIONS
CashApp: $miadibes
ZELLE: (404)980-4330 KELLY MAHFOOD
Go Fund Me: gofund.me/cbe0c6b4
email: miadibes@gmail.com

12

What We Gained

Lessons in Leadership, Humility, and Resilience

The journey to Mount Prospect gave us more than we ever anticipated. It taught us how to lead through uncertainty, how to serve with humility, and how to bounce back when plans fell apart. From every late-evening Zoom meeting to every challenge we overcame on-site, we walked away stronger and more grounded in our purpose.

We learned that leadership isn't about having all the answers—it's about showing up, listening deeply, and adapting when things go off-script. We leaned on each other's strengths and learned to trust the process, even when the path wasn't clear.

The Power of Community Collaboration

This mission confirmed something we always believed: **community is the most powerful force for change.** The health fair was only possible because of collaboration. From local churches and businesses to international volunteers and donors, everyone played a role in the movement. We watched people come together—not for credit, but for love. That kind of unity doesn't just create impact—it builds legacy.

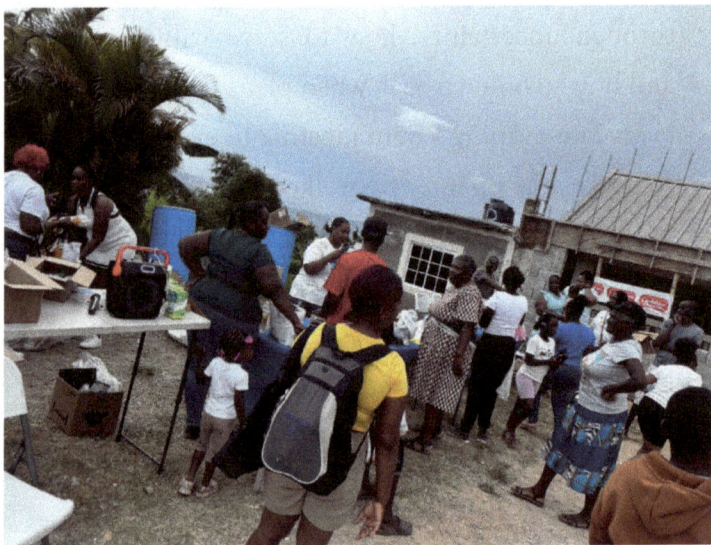

Cleaning up after the event

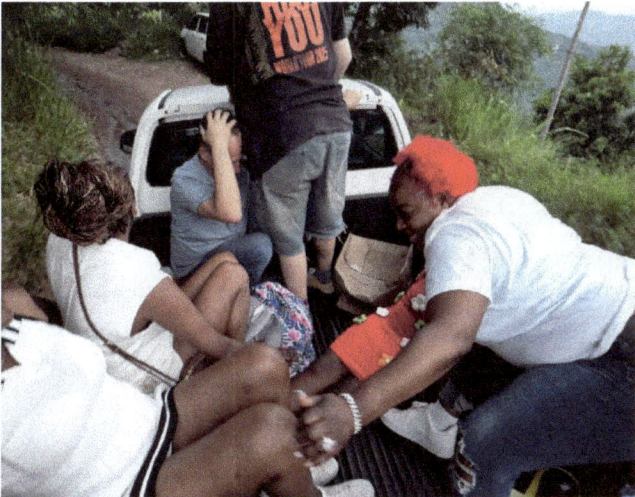

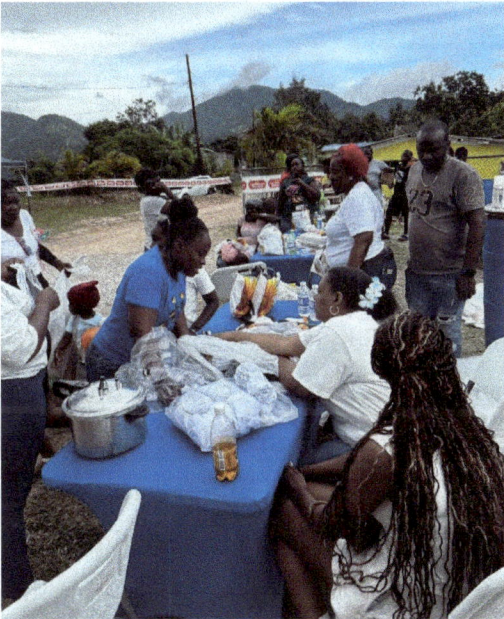

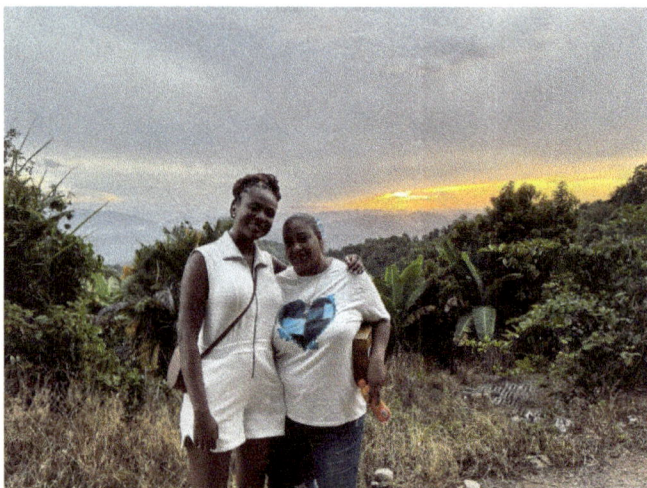

Kelly and Shannon after the health fair

Evaluation and Post-Event Feedback

After the fair, we took time to reflect and evaluate. We collected feedback from volunteers, community members, and healthcare partners. What worked? What didn't? What surprised us?

There were common themes: appreciation for the organized flow, gratitude for the services provided, and a desire for even more access to medical professionals and screenings next time. These insights weren't just noted—they became the blueprint for future planning.

13

What Comes Next

Planning for 2026 and Scaling Miadibes Cares

With the 2025 health fair behind us, our eyes are set on **2026—and beyond**. Planning has already begun for the **Second Annual Mount Prospect Health Fair**, with early goals to double the number of attendees, expand services to include dental and mental health care, and enhance follow-up care through local partnerships.

But Miadibes Cares isn't just about one health fair. We are beginning to dream bigger—health education workshops, mobile clinics, outreach into other underserved communities in Jamaica, and possibly launching a Youth Health Ambassador Program.

Nonprofit Growth Strategy

To make this vision sustainable, we are refining our **nonprofit infrastructure**. This includes:

- Finalizing our 501(c)(3) and Jamaican charitable status
- Building a diverse Board of Directors
- Securing multi-year funding through grants, donors, and corporate partners
- Creating a volunteer pipeline with training and mentorship programs
- Implementing better tracking systems to measure outcomes and impact

We know growth won't be easy—but we're committed to it. Because the need is great. And our mission is greater.

How to Keep Momentum Going

Momentum is a fragile thing—it must be nurtured with intention. For Miadibes Cares, that means **staying rooted in community**, **keeping our "why" front and center**, and continuing to **celebrate small wins along the way.**

Whether hosting local fundraising events, sharing monthly impact updates on social media, or organizing reunion calls with our volunteers, we're building systems of encouragement and accountability.

We believe this is just the beginning of a movement that will bring **health, healing, and hope** to generations.

The next move is our award ceremony. Miadibes Cares Awards Ceremony Gala. It will be a black and white formal affair. It will be held on the evening of Friday, June, 12th, 2026.

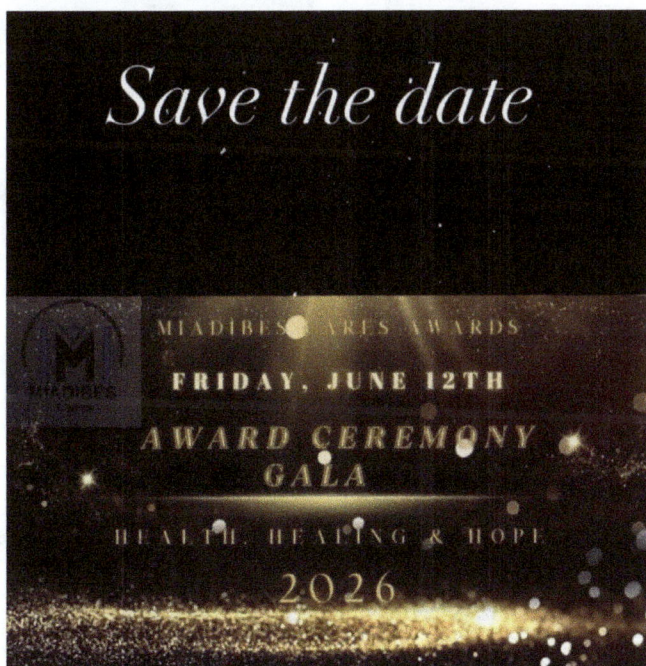

14

A Blueprint for Change

How-To for Organizing a Rural Health Fair

If Miadibes Cares has taught us anything, it's that **ordinary people can create extraordinary change**. This chapter is for anyone who feels called to serve but doesn't know where to start. Here's what we learned, step by step.

1. **Start with the Why**

   Identify the need. Talk to the community. Understand what's missing and who is most impacted. Your "why" is your anchor—it will guide every decision.

2. **Build a Core Team**

   You can't do it alone. Surround yourself with people who are dependable, passionate, and diverse in skill sets. Weekly meetings and a shared vision are essential.

3. **Secure a Location and Date Early**

Especially in rural areas, infrastructure can be limited. Visit the site in person, evaluate accessibility, and confirm permissions well in advance.

4. **Develop a Proposal and Budget**

Outline your goals, expected outcomes, logistics, and a detailed budget. Include categories for medical supplies, volunteer support, marketing, security, transportation, and contingencies.

5. **Engage the Community from the Start**

Involve local leaders, churches, schools, and residents in the planning process. Their support will be your foundation.

6. **Begin Fundraising Early**

Use every tool available: GoFundMe, community events, corporate sponsorships, and social media campaigns. Be transparent and consistent in your updates.

7. **Handle Logistics with Care**

Barrels and shipments take time. Plan around customs fees and transport issues. Designate team leads for each major area: medical services, volunteer coordination, hospitality, registration, etc.

8. **Create a Day-Of Timeline and Roles**

Draft a minute-by-minute agenda for the health fair. Assign clear roles and provide walkie-talkies or WhatsApp groups to manage communication.

9. **Collect Data and Feedback**

Capture how many people were served, what services were provided, and community testimonials. This information is vital for credibility, reporting, and future funding.

10. **Celebrate and Reflect**

Take time to thank your team and recognize their hard work. Host a debrief session, document lessons learned and share your success with supporters.

Sample Budgets, Templates, Sponsor Letters

To make this chapter truly actionable, we've included:

- A **sample rural health fair budget**
- A **volunteer sign-up template**
- A **basic project timeline**
- Two **sponsorship request letter templates**
- A **thank-you letter for donors and partners**
- A **post-event evaluation form**

These resources are free to adapt and share—because change multiplies when we lift each other up.

Building Your Own Mission from Scratch

You don't need to be a nonprofit expert to start something powerful. You just need vision, heart, and a little help.

Start where you are. Use what you have. Partner with people who share your passion. And don't wait for everything to be perfect. If we had waited, Miadibes Cares would still be a dream instead of a legacy in the making.

Let this be your **invitation to build**, to serve, and to dream aloud.

You are more ready than you think.

Appendices

Available online at https://www.miadibescares.org

A. Full 2025 Health Fair Budget (JMD/USD Conversion)
B. Sample Sponsor Letter & Recognition Tiers
C. Volunteer Job Descriptions
D. Policies: Consent, Data, Diversity & Risk
E. Mission Trip Itinerary 2025–2026
F. Testimonials from Residents & Volunteers

About the Author

Kelly Mahfood is a seasoned nurse, dedicated caregiver, and the passionate founder of **Miadibes Cares**, a nonprofit organization devoted to improving healthcare access in underserved communities—starting with her beloved Jamaica in the town her grandmother resides, Mount Prospect.

With over 25 years of experience in nursing, Kelly has worked across various healthcare settings, bringing compassion, leadership, and a strong sense of purpose to every role. Her deep roots in Maryland, New York, Georgia and Jamaica inspired her to launch Miadibes Cares, blending her clinical expertise with a lifelong mission of service.

Kelly is more than a nurse, she's a visionary. Her commitment to uplifting others through health, education, and community empowerment came to life during the Miadibes Cares inaugural mission trip to Mount Prospect, Jamaica in June 2025. This book is a reflection of that journey: the challenges, the breakthroughs, and the powerful connections made along the way.

When she's not coordinating health fairs or mentoring future healthcare leaders, Kelly enjoys spending time with her family, tackling one of her many DIY projects, traveling, and dreaming up new ways to serve those who need it most.

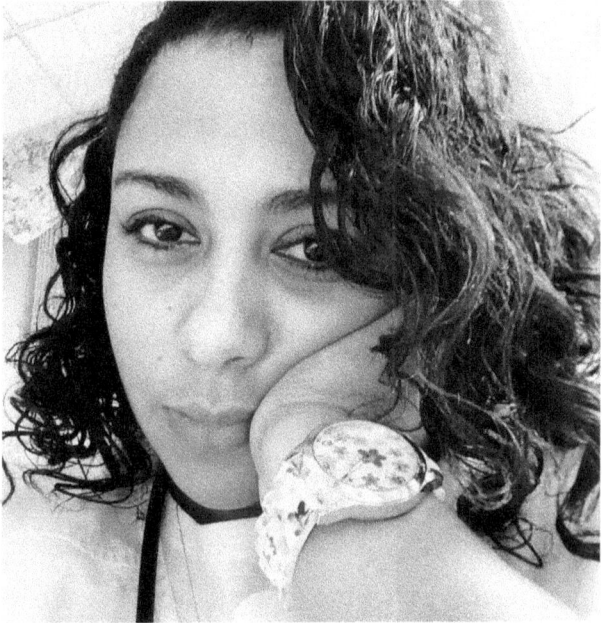

www.ingramcontent.com/pod-product-compliance
Lightning Source LLC
Chambersburg PA
CBHW070911280326
41934CB00008B/1669